Nursing & Health Survival Guide

Record Keeping

Pauline Merrix
Sue Lillyman

Routledge
Taylor & Francis Group

LONDON AND NEW YORK

T0186506

First published 2012 by Pearson Education Limited

Published 2014 by Routledge
2 Park Square, Milton Park, Abingdon, Oxon OX14 4RN
711 Third Avenue, New York, NY 10017, USA

Routledge is an imprint of the Taylor & Francis Group, an informa business

Copyright © 2012, Taylor & Francis.

Notices
Knowledge and best practice in this field are constantly changing. As new research and experie broaden our understanding, changes in research methods, professional practices, or medical treatment may become necessary.

Practitioners and researchers must always rely on their own experience and knowledge in evaluating and using any information, methods, compounds, or experiments described herein. I using such information or methods they should be mindful of their own safety and the safety of others, including parties for whom they have a professional responsibility.

To the fullest extent of the law, neither the Publisher nor the authors, contributors, or editors, assume any liability for any injury and/or damage to persons or property as a matter of products liability, negligence or otherwise, or from any use or operation of any methods, products, instructions, or ideas contained in the material herein.

ISBN 13: 978-0-273-76064-1 (hbk)

British Library Cataloguing-in-Publication Data
A catalogue record for this book is available from the British Library

Library of Congress Cataloging-in-Publication Data
Merrix, Pauline.
    Record keeping / Pauline Merrix, Sue Lillyman.
      p. ; cm. -- (Nursing & health survival guide)
    Includes bibliographical references.
    ISBN 978-0-273-76064-1
    I. Lillyman, Sue. II. Title. III. Series: Nursing & health survival guides.
    [DNLM: 1. Nursing Records--Great Britain--Handbooks. 2. Forms and Records Control--methods--Great Britain--Handbooks. WY 49]

    610.68--dc23
                                                                      2012005224
Typeset in 8/9.5pt Helvetica by 35

contents

Record keeping is an integral part in the delivery of healthcare and should be considered a tool of professional practice. All NHS records are public records and come under the terms of the Public Records Act 1958 and Data Protection Act of 1998.

The Data Protection Act 1998 defines a health record as:

'consisting of information about the physical or mental health or condition of an identifiable individual made by or on behalf of a health professional in connection with the care of that individual.'

Effective record keeping is a sign of a safe and skilled practitioner and as such requires practice and continual development. It should not be considered as an optional extra that can be fitted in when time allows.

Record keeping and communication are included in most professional codes of conduct including those of the Nursing and Midwifery Council and the Health Professional Council. The codes require you to keep clear and accurate records of the discussions you have, the assessments you make, the treatment and medicines you give and how effective these have been.

Record keeping continues to be an issue within practice. It has been raised within the Robert Francis Inquiry Report into Mid Staffordshire NHS Trust (2010) and remains the fourth most common allegation in fitness for practice cases seen by the Nursing and Midwifery Council as identified in their annual report. Other professional bodies also continue to see cases of professional misconduct in relation to record keeping.

'Not having time is no longer acceptable as professional bodies consider accurate record keeping as one of their requirements in maintaining a practitioner's fitness to practice.'

Currently there is no single model for documenting patient health records but all National Health Service Trusts will have guidance on recording, handling and storage of records. This can be found within the trust clinical governance framework and should be read in conjunction with this book.

As well as looking at the record keeping required by qualified practitioners, this book will consider record keeping undertaken by students in their practice placement records, patient/service-user health records and other records kept by patients and professionals.

The themes of patient confidentiality, recording patient consent and the professional accountability of the practitioner can all be demonstrated through effective record keeping and will also be discussed.

Records

As noted in the introduction a health record is:

- A permanent form of information relating to an individual's physical or mental health
- A record where the individual can be identified from that information
- Made by a health professional in connection with the care of that individual

The Records Management NHS Code of Practice (2006) states that all practitioners working within the NHS are responsible for any records they create or use whilst caring for an individual. These documents are then public records.

Records that identify a living individual are referred to as **personal data**. These can also include information where a person can be identified from the data in conjunction with other data/information that the professional holds.

This can include:

- Name
- Address
- Age
- Race
- Religion
- Gender
- Physical health
- Mental health
- Sexual health

■ WHY ARE RECORDS NEEDED?

Good records are needed in order to:

- Communicate information to other professionals and facilitate continuity of care
- Keep a record of the day to day care given to patients
- Provide a chronological account of the patient's life, illnesses
- Identify who did what and to what effect for the patient
- Enable early detection of changes in the patient's condition
- Evaluate the patient's progress
- Enable patients to have greater involvement in their care and demonstrate a patient centred approach to the care received
- Demonstrate patient safety and quality of care
- Demonstrate professional accountability
- Support clinical audit and clinical governance
- Inform medico-legal investigations and aid in the management of enquiries and complaints
- Inform research

■ TYPES OF RECORDS

The Records Management NHS Code of Practice (2006) suggests there are a number of different forms of records; these may include:
- Handwritten or electronic clinical notes
- A&E, birth and all other registers
- Theatre registers and minor operations lists
- Patient/parent held records
- Emails
- Letters to and from other health professionals
- Laboratory reports
- Radiographs and other imaging reports and outputs and images

- Printouts from monitoring equipment
- Incident reports and statements
- Photographs/slides and other images
- Microfilms
- Videos
- Tape-recordings, video and cassettes
- Text messages
- Scanned records

■ WHAT MAKES A GOOD RECORD?

- Clearly identified patient/service-user name
- Arranged in chronological order with the most recent on top
- Legible handwriting
- Entries signed with the nurse's name and job title printed alongside the first entry
- Student's entry countersigned by a qualified practitioner
- Made as near to the time of the episode of care as possible and before the relevant staff member goes off duty. (This fulfils the legal requirement that records are contemporaneous.)
- Accurate and recorded in such a way that the meaning is clear and easy to understand
- Factual and do not include unnecessary abbreviations
- Facilitates communication in a full and effective way with other professions, ensuring they have all the information they need about people in your care
- Changes to entries follow set procedures
- Readable when photocopied or scanned. (The use of black ink is best.)
- Based on professional judgements (see below)

- Objective
- Written so as to be compliant with the Race Relations Act (1976) and Disability Discrimination Act (2005)

■ WHAT MAKES A POOR RECORD?

- Inaccurate information
- Illegible and poorly structured writing
- Subjective comments that cannot be supported by facts and accompanied by irrelevant or offensive speculations
- Unauthorised or retrospective changes to the record
- The use of sarcasm or humorous abbreviations to describe patients in your care. (These could be viewed as disrespectful comments.)
- Notes that are not comprehensive enough, with omissions or gaps in the record
- Anonymised recordings
- Jargon and unnecessary abbreviations

■ RECORDING PROFESSIONAL JUDGEMENTS

Including professional judgements should help you to decide what is relevant and should be recorded.

These should include:

- Use of evidence based methods of assessment and reviews
- Critical thinking in relation to care given
- Evidence based practice for diagnosing and care planning
- High quality information that justifies the approach to care taken
- Information received and given to the patient about their care and treatment

- Risks or problems that have arisen with the action taken to deal with them
- Informed consent gained, explicit or implied, ensuring an entry is made if consent is withheld by the patient and the reasons for this
- Identifying the outcome of care given

■ BEING OBJECTIVE IN YOUR RECORDS

Objectivity is another important feature of good record keeping. State facts from what you see, feel, hear and smell. By recording these four sensory observations you are attempting to distinguish between **fact** (objectivity), which is what actually happened, and **opinion** (subjectivity), which is what might have happened.

Examples of what you **See**:
- Bleeding, urine colour, pallor, sweating, deformities, bruises, oedema, sores/lesions, redness, body fluid colour, pupil reaction

Examples of what you **Feel** (to the touch):
- Crepitus, dampness, localised heat/cold, pulses

Examples of what you **Hear**:
- Complaints, moaning, breathing, heart sounds

Examples of what you **Smell**:
- Faecal odours, fruity odours, foul smelling drainage, and alcohol breath

Examples of **Objective, factual statements**:
- No complaints or pain or discomfort
- Eyes closed and respirations regular

- Thrashing about in bed
- I.V. Dextrose 5% infusing at 60 drops per minute with site clear and no redness

Examples of **Subjective statements**:
- Had a good day
- Usual night
- Appears restless
- I.V. running well

■ USING ABBREVIATIONS

The use of abbreviations is discouraged by the Nursing and Midwifery Council and other professional bodies as they can prove difficult for patients/service-users to understand. In addition, they can be misinterpreted by other professions. If abbreviations are used in a record there must be an accompanying glossary which has been approved by the appropriate professional body or the NHS local Trust.

■ HOW TO AMEND ENTRIES IF NEEDED

- Alterations must be accompanied by your name, job title and with a signature and date alongside the alteration.
- The use of Tippex or similar correcting techniques is strongly discouraged.
- The original record, as well as the alteration, must be clear and auditable.

■ ELECTRONIC RECORDS

When creating and using electronic records you must:

- Password protect any files/computers
- Always log-out of any computer system when work on it is finished
- Never leave a terminal unattended and still logged in
- Not share logins with other people
- Not reveal passwords to others
- Always clear the screen of a patient's information before viewing another
- Ensure entries you make in electronic records are clearly attributable to you
- Abide by the Data Protection Act 1998

■ STORAGE OF RECORDS

The Secretary of State for Health and all NHS organisations have a duty under the Public Records Act 2005 to make arrangements for safe keeping of records. There is an appointed 'Keeper of Records' who is answerable to parliament. Within the Trusts the chief executives and senior managers are personally accountable for the management of records within their organisation. All individuals who work within the NHS are responsible for the records that they produce.

To meet legal requirements:
- Adult records must be kept for at least 8 years
- Paediatric and maternity records for at least 25 years
- Psychiatric notes up to 20 years
- General health records 8 years after the conclusion of treatment or death

The storage of records is an important feature of the record keeping process. Records must be returned to locked storage as soon as possible and should not be left in offices, cars or individual homes. You should not leave computer records on screens where they might be viewed by unauthorised staff or members of the public.

■ PATIENT HELD RECORDS

Patient held records were first introduced in the National Health Service in 2001 following a recommendation made in the National Service Framework for Older People. Within this system, the patient has custody of their records for on-going care but the records will eventually be stored with the National Health Service when treatment is no longer required or the patient dies. Parent and patient held records are currently confined to use in the midwifery and primary care services.

■ DESTRUCTION OF RECORDS (shredding or incineration)

Before any destruction takes place it must be ensured that:
- Actions are clearly minuted by the appropriate personnel. This could be a records committee or relevant health professional body
- Confidentiality is maintained
- The value of the records for long term research has been assessed

Unofficial destruction of records by any health care professional is a serious matter that can result in disciplinary procedure.

Access to records

■ FOR THE PATIENT

There is a formal procedure for patients to apply for their records.

The Data Protection Act of 1998 makes provision for the regulation of the processing of information for a living individual held by their GP, optician or hospital.

There is nothing in law to prevent a professional showing a patient their records. Equally when an individual is requesting a copy of their records there is no obligation to give a reason if the access is denied. Refusal, however, should be if it is believed that by releasing the record the information would cause serious physical or mental harm to the person or others.

Once requested, the records should be given within 40 days but best practice is within 21 days. There is usually a fee.

■ TO SOLICITORS

Under the Department of Health Code of Practice: Confidentiality (2003) information given to solicitors should be with full understanding and explicit consent gained from the individual patient. It will include only limited information that is relevant to the reason information is being sought.

■ TO THE COURT

Information given can include only information that is limited to the terms of the order.

■ TO THE POLICE

There is no general right for the police to access health records. As there is no statute which regulates disclosure to the police, information can be given with explicit consent from the patient or if there is a robust public interest justification. The information should be limited to meet the need asked for. The patient must be informed of the disclosure unless it will defeat the object of the investigation, allow a potential criminal to escape or put staff or others at risk.

■ TO THE MEDIA

There is no basis for disclosure to the media. In exceptional circumstances, with consent obtained or 'exceptional' public interest there might be a case for disclosure. This is usually given through an appointed Trust spokesperson.

■ FOR RESEARCH

If possible research should include anonymised records, otherwise explicit consent is required. (Ethical approval for access to records is covered later in this book.)

■ FOR A STUDENT

The Nursing and Midwifery Council gives the following advice on accessing records:
- If as a student you have problems with missing notes or problems accessing records you must report the matter to someone in authority or seek advice from your mentor or tutor.
- If as a student you are involved in, or participate in, research ensure you follow the University and clinical

provider guidance and policy on ethics governing research and seek extra guidance from your mentor or tutor if necessary.

• You should not access the record of any person, or their family, to find out personal information that is not relevant to their care.

■ AFTER DEATH

Once an individual is deceased the Access to Health Records Act 1990 governs access to their health records.

Preparing for the legal defensibility of record keeping

The resolution of clinical disputes can be dealt with quickly and efficiently by well written, accurate, factual and consistent records and may not need to be referred to the National Health Service complaints procedure. However, records are considered legal documents and as such can be used as evidence in a Court of Law in cases of clinical negligence. Patient/service-user records may also be called as evidence by any professional governing body in a case of a practitioner's fitness to practice.

If a practitioner is summoned as a witness in a court case they must give evidence. It may be that the incident in question was a considerable time ago. A complaint can be made up to 12 months following the episode of care; however, it is at the discretion of the complaints manager if over this period so therefore can be even older. In such cases it may be difficult for you to remember the patient and the care that you provided, so the health record is vital and presents an accurate record of your actions and hence your evidence to the court.

To ensure good practice with record keeping and to aid the courts or hearing committees, the guide below should be followed. These points should be considered along with the section **What makes a good record**?

- Do not leave the writing of records for later – you may forget something that may prove important at a later date.
- Ensure you make contemporaneous records – this can be defined as recordings made in the clinical notes as near to the time of the care giving event as possible. For example: An entry in the notes three days after the actual care has been given is not considered to be a contemporaneous record so in a court of law the records could be questioned as to their reliability as a true and accurate account of what has occurred. Without a contemporaneous record you may be challenged as to whether you have done what you claim to have done.
- Detail every point in a chronological order – treat each entry as if it were a step-by-step journey.
- Do not write anything that you would not be happy to repeat in a court of law.
- Keep notes clean and tidy.
- Date, time and sign all entries – cross-examination by lawyers often concentrates on the beginnings and endings of entries in order to gain a full and accurate representation of events.
- Distinguish fact from opinion, record objectively and avoid subjective comments – the two are often confused when people are writing records. In court the 'what happened' or objective recordings are very important.

- Use black ink to ensure any photocopying is easy to read.
- Do not attribute negligence or blame to other staff, patients, their relatives, friends or carers.
- Always record consent carefully.
- Ensure pages are numbered. It is more difficult for pages to be removed covertly.
- Ensure your practice is current and up to date, using evidence based practice.

Confidentiality

■ IN RECORDS OR CONVERSATIONS

Confidentiality is a fundamental part of professional practice that protects human rights. This is identified in Article 8 of the European Convention on Human Rights 1966 which states:

Everyone has the right to respect for his private and family life, his home and his correspondence.

A duty of confidence arises when one person discloses information to another. For example: A patient tells a clinician something about themselves. In this situation it is reasonable to expect that the information will be held in confidence. The Department of Health states in the NHS Confidentiality Code of Practice 2003 that this is:

- A legal obligation derived from case law
- A requirement established within professional codes of conduct
- Included within the National Health Service employment contracts as a specific requirement linked to disciplinary procedures

All healthcare practitioners owe a duty of confidentiality and a duty to ensure that material of a personal and confidential nature is treated with the appropriate degree of security. Any such breach of confidence may lead to a patient lodging a complaint under the National Health Service complaints procedure.

This includes not gossiping about individuals in your care and taking care if discussing cases in public areas.

■ FOR COURSE WORK

If you are a student on any course **you must** make anonymous any information in your coursework or assessment documentation that may directly or indirectly identify patients/service-users, staff, relatives, carers or clinical placement providers. You should ensure you have gained informed consent prior to including the anonymised information.

Compliance with the Data Protection Act of 1998 and common law of confidentially should satisfy the human rights requirements.

The Nursing and Midwifery Council further advises on confidentiality that:
- You need to be fully aware of the legal requirements and guidance regarding confidentiality. The common law of confidentiality expects that information given to a nurse/midwife is only used for the purpose for which it was given and will not be discussed without permission.
- You should be aware of the rules governing confidentiality in respect of the supply and use of data for secondary purposes.
- You should not discuss the people in your care in places where you might be overheard.

■ THE CALDICOTT REPORT

A review was commissioned in 1997 by the Chief Medical Officer of England owing to the increasing concern about patient information and the development of information technology in the National Health Service. Following the report of a committee chaired by Dame Fiona Caldicott each National Health Service organisation had to appoint a Caldicott Guardian.

These are senior health professionals, usually at Trust board level, who are responsible for protecting the confidentiality of patient/service-user information and enabling appropriate information sharing.

The Guardian advises on the legal and ethical processing of information. The mandate issued from the Department of Health in 1999 covers all organisations that have access to patient records. This includes acute trusts, ambulance trusts, mental health trusts, primary care trusts, strategic health authorities, and special health authorities such as NHS Direct.

Caldicott Guardians were introduced into social care in 2002. The role is particularly important with the implementation of the National Programme for Information Technology and Common Assessment Frameworks, where health and social care professionals work closely and appropriate sharing of patient information is essential.

■ CALDICOTT KEY PRINCIPLES

- Justify the purpose of using confidential information. Every proposed use or transfer of patient identifiable information within or outside of the organisation should be clearly defined and scrutinised, with continuing uses regularly reviewed, by 'an appropriate guardian'.

- Do not use patient identifiable information unless it is absolutely necessary. The need for patient identification should be reviewed regularly.
- Use the minimum necessary patient identifiable information.
- Access to patient identifiable information should be on a strict need to know basis.
- Everyone should be aware of their responsibilities and respect patient confidentiality.
- Understand and comply with the law.

Further information can be found in the Caldicott Guardian pages on the Department of Health website.

All staff working in the health care setting may need to seek advice from a Caldicott Guardian if they are unsure of any element of care involving the use of confidential information and disclosure.

■ DISCLOSURE

Disclosure means the giving of information. There are circumstances where disclosure of information is desirable but this should be accompanied by lawful and ethical considerations.

- Disclosure is only lawful and ethical if the individual has given consent to the information being passed on.
- Such consent must be freely and fully given.

As a practitioner, if you think there has been a breach of confidentiality due to an individual's behaviour or as a result of organisational systems failure then you must act without delay if you believe a colleague or anyone else may be putting someone at risk. This can be by informing your line manager or if you are a student your mentor, tutor or a qualified senior person. You have a professional duty to take action to ensure the people in your care are protected and failure to take such action could amount to professional misconduct.

■ CONSENT TO DISCLOSURE

Consent to disclosure of confidential information may be:

- Explicit consent:
  This is obtained when the person in the care of a practitioner agrees to the disclosure and has been informed of the reason for that disclosure and with whom the information may or will be shared. Explicit consent can be written or spoken.

- Implied consent:
  This is obtained when it is assumed the person in your care understands their information may be shared within the healthcare team. Health care practitioners should make the people in their care aware of this routine sharing of information and clearly record in the patient/client notes any objections.

- Disclosure without consent:
  The Law, by using common law, allows healthcare staff to disclose personal information in order to prevent and support detection, investigation and punishment of serious crime and/or to prevent abuse or serious harm to others.

For example:
○ Disclosing information in relation to crimes against the person concerning rape, child abuse, murder, kidnapping or injuries sustained from knife or gunshot wounds.
○ Capable of justification by reason of the public interest: The term public interest describes the exceptional circumstances that justify overruling the right of an individual to confidentiality in order to serve a broader social concern. This could involve cases of misconduct and illegality.

(See examples of scenarios 1–3 at the end of the book.)

Consent to treatment and record keeping

Treatment and care given without patient/service-user consent is considered in law to be assault. Gaining and documenting consent when it has been given is a vital part of the defence against assault. It is because the issue of consent is so important that the gaining and recording of consent must be rigorous, transparent and demonstrate a clear level of professional accountability. All discussions and decisions relating to consent must be recorded accurately.

The Nursing and Midwifery Council gives the following advice regarding students and consent:
- If you are a student you must make sure people know this and respect the right for patients/service-users to request care to be given by a registered professional.
- You must ensure that you gain consent before you begin any treatment or care.

- You must respect and support people's rights to accept or decline treatment and care.
- You must be aware of the legislation regarding mental capacity.

Patients have a legal and ethical right to determine what happens to their bodies. No adult or child, competent to make his own medical decisions may be given medical treatment without his consent. However, seeking consent may be difficult either because of patients' disabilities or because they have difficulty fully understanding (capacity) and, in addition, difficulty in communicating their decision. Before anyone can give a valid consent to treatment he/she must possess the requisite capacity. The Mental Capacity Act 2005 states that there is a presumption that every person has capacity to consent to or refuse medical treatment unless it is proved otherwise.

■ HOW TO ASSESS COMPETENCE/CAPACITY

For a patient/service-user to have the capacity to take a particular decision, they must be able to:

- Comprehend and retain information material to the decision, especially as to the consequences of having or not having treatment
- Use and weigh this information in the decision-making process

In order for patients/service-users to give valid consent it must be given voluntarily, not under duress, and they must be given quality and relevant information to ensure it is informed consent.

■ WHAT TO RECORD IN THE HEALTH RECORDS CONCERNING CONSENT

- The date consent has been given
- The type of consent: implied, verbal or written
- If consent is withheld or withdrawn during treatment, the discussions and reasons given by the patient
- Any changes in the type of consent during the treatment
- Consent involving children must be comprehensive and state any discussions with parents or adults who have parental responsibility
- Any formal written consent form signed by the patient/service-user

■ CHILDREN AND CONSENT

16–17 years of age – Once children reach the age of 16, they are presumed in law to be competent to give consent for themselves for their own medical care. However, it is good practice to encourage children to involve their families in decision-making. Where a competent child does ask you to keep confidence, you must do so, unless you can justify disclosure on the grounds that you have reasonable cause to suspect that the child is suffering, or is likely to suffer significant harm. You should however seek to persuade them to involve their family, unless you believe that it is not in their best interests to do so.

Under 16 – Unlike 16 or 17 year olds, children under the age of 16 are not automatically presumed to be legally competent to make decisions about their health care. However, the courts have stated that under 16s will be competent to give valid consent to health care if they have sufficient understanding and intelligence to enable them to understand fully what is proposed. Therefore those who have the capacity to understand and make decisions about their treatment have the same rights in relation to giving confidential information.

This includes giving information to parents where the child has disclosed information in confidence to the practitioner (see scenario at the end of the book).

■ LOSS OF CAPACITY

In relation to confidentially and record information if an individual has lost capacity and there is no advanced care directive then best interest is used.

■ CONSENT: DISABILITY DISCRIMINATION ACT

Competence to consent should not breach the Disability Discrimination Act of 1995 and therefore information should be provided in various formats for different disabilities.

■ RIGHT TO WITHDRAW/REFUSE CONSENT

Everyone has the right to withdraw consent at any time for treatment and the use and/or disclosure of their personal information. This may include the right to refuse to allow other professionals to view the health records. If the individual refuses their information to be shared with other professionals then it should be explained that this might affect the quality of their care and services. This should be documented.

Ethics, accountability and record keeping

Ethics can be viewed as the professional morals that we as healthcare professionals support and can be considered within the following seven principles:

- **Autonomy**: the individual has a right to be self-governing
- **Beneficence**: the well-being or benefit of the individual should be promoted
- **Non-malfeasance**: do no harm
- **Justice**: equals are considered equally
- **Veracity**: telling the truth
- **Confidentiality**: the protection of the patient's right to privacy
- **Fidelity**: the principle of faithfulness and keeping promises

It should be clear from this list which of these ethical principles has direct links to record keeping. However, all of these principles are linked to the delivery of health care, the recording of the care given, the maintaining of patient confidentiality and the professional accountability of the practitioner.

Accountability can be defined as the requirement that each practitioner is answerable and responsible for the outcome of his or her professional actions.

The Nursing and Midwifery Council states:

'As a professional, you are personally accountable for actions and omissions in your practice and must always be able to justify your decisions.'

As a professional you are accountable to:

- **The public** – through criminal law
- **The employer** – through contract law
- **The patient/service-user** – through a duty of care and the common law of negligence and through civil law
- **The profession** – through the Codes which includes standards of conduct, performance and ethics

These four principal applications of accountability all relate to, and are dependent, in part, on the practitioner's record keeping skills. One way of demonstrating accountability is through the recording of your actions. Patient/service-user health records remain the most tangible evidence of a professional practitioner's practice and are your main defence if assessments or decisions are ever scrutinised. With the development and growing autonomy within some areas of health care, the specialist practitioners can often feel their accountability to be greater than that of the traditional role of the practitioner. Because of this, they may wish to devise documentation specific to their speciality.

When acting as a mentor, the registered practitioner must recognise his/her accountability for entries to records made by students or others under their supervision by reading and counter-signing the entry.

Maintaining your skills for record keeping

The professional bodies' codes of professional conduct require all practitioners to maintain and update their knowledge and skills in order to remain on the professional register. Each practitioner has a joint obligation, with the employer, to develop and maintain the appropriate level of skills and awareness of best practice required for effective record keeping. This can be achieved in many ways. For example:

- Monitoring record keeping skills by regular auditing of records. Self or peer auditing, using a tool, is not time consuming and should be considered as an effective, non-threatening and credible method of reviewing record keeping practice. (Figure 1 gives a typical example of an audit tool.)
- Incident reporting involving record keeping errors.
- Clinical supervision using record keeping problems to prompt group or individual discussions.
- Reflection.

These are all ways of maintaining competence and confidence in the skills required for effective record keeping. These techniques cannot be underestimated in their importance in achieving clear, concise contemporaneous notes that serve primarily to enhance patient care but are also essential in protecting the professional practice.

Figure 1 Tool for auditing health records

AUDIT CRITERIA	YES	NO	N/A	COMMENTS
Is the patient/service-user's name on the records?				
Are all the entries signed and accompanied by evidence of the full name and professional status?				
Where an unqualified person has written in the record, have their entries been countersigned by the registrant who delegated the task?				
Are all written entries legible?				
Are all entries contemporaneous?				
If any entries have been crossed out, are they still legible and accompanied by name, job title, date and signature?				
Is the documentation free of correcting fluid?				
If any clinical abbreviations are used, is there an accompanying glossary?				
Is the record arranged in chronological order with the most recent on top?				

Figure 1 (*continued*)

AUDIT CRITERIA	YES	NO	N/A	COMMENTS
Does the record show the stages of assessment, planning and implementing care, evaluation of care and evidence based practice?				
Where patient consent has been obtained, is it clearly recorded?				

Relevant legislation

You should be aware of the following pieces of legislation relating to confidentiality.

- **The Data Protection Act 1998**
  This Act governs the processing of information that identifies living individuals. Processing includes holding, recording, using and disclosing of information. This Act applies to all forms of media, including paper and electronic in both National Health Service and the private sector.
- **The Human Fertilisation and Embryology Act 1990**
  This Act regulates the provision of new reproductive technology services and places a statutory ban upon the disclosure of information concerning gamete donors and people receiving treatment under the Act. Unauthorised disclosure of such information by healthcare professionals and others has been made a criminal offence.

- **The National Health Service Venereal Disease Regulation 1974**
  This states that health authorities should take all necessary steps to ensure that identifiable information relating to persons being treated for sexually transmitted diseases should not be disclosed.
- **The Mental Capacity Act 2005**
  This provides a legal framework to empower and protect people who may lack capacity to make some decisions for themselves. The assessor of an 'individual's capacity to make a decision will usually be the person who is directly concerned with the individual at the time the decision needs to be made', and may be a different health worker or social care worker at varying times when different capacity decisions are being made.
- **The Freedom of Information Act 2000**
  This Act grants people right of access to information that is not covered by the Data Protection Act 1998. For example: Information which does not contain a person's identifiable details.
- **The Computer Misuse Act 1990**
  This Act secures computer programs and data against unauthorised access or alteration.
- **The Access to Health Records Act 1990**
  This provides supplementary right, in addition to the Data Protection Act 1998 for extracts or copies by the holder of health records, to patients. If the record is over forty days old a fee may be levied. If the record is less than forty days there is no charge.

Other records

■ PATIENT'S ADVANCE STATEMENT

An advance statement can be written or expressed wishes of the patient declaring what they would, or would not, like to happen in the event of their condition deteriorating and capacity being lost. This might include where they might wish to be cared for and preferred place of death and their funeral choices. These are documents created by the patient but will include personal information.

■ ADVANCE DECISION (previously known as living wills or advance directives)

This is a written document created again by the individual that states what treatment or life sustaining treatment they wish to refuse. It is a legally binding declaration of the individual's choice to refuse certain treatments, some of which may be life sustaining treatments, in anticipation of how their condition may affect them in the future at a time when they do not have the capacity to make these decisions themselves. These documents are written and kept by the individual but may be brought into hospital with them. These records come into force once the patient loses capacity to make a decision at the time. They should be handled the same as any other documentation.

■ PERSONAL PROFESSIONAL RECORDS

These are records made by the practitioner for their own professional development. These might include a portfolio for their professional body or to demonstrate

their achievement for the Knowledge and Skills Framework
or a personal reflective log or diary. All these should not
contain any patient information and should be treated
as any other documentation in relation to storage and
confidentiality.

Conclusion

All records and patient's information given by an individual
should be treated with respect and confidentially. Records
that are created by the professional should also be of a high
standard in order to deliver a high standard of care to that
individual.

■ SCENARIOS FROM THE DEPARTMENT OF HEALTH CONFIDENTIALITY: NHS CODE OF PRACTICE (2003) DEMONSTRATING PUBLIC INTEREST DISCLOSURE

Scenario 1

A receptionist at a GP surgery sees a patient leave
the building and get into his car. On driving from the
car park, the patient's car collides with and damages
another patient's car. The driver does not stop, believing
that nobody has seen the incident and instead drives
away without leaving his details. Through her role at
the surgery, the receptionist knows the identity of the
patient.

Can the receptionist report the crime? What details
can the receptionist provide about the accident and
the driver?

Decision

A minor crime has been committed, but no serious crime or serious harm done. Therefore there is insufficient public interest justification for revealing confidential patient information (for example: from within the patient's case notes; or even the fact that the patient has attended the surgery). However, a crime has been committed and the receptionist would be entitled to report the incident, including the identity of the patient, to the police, but should not reveal confidential patient information.

Scenario 2

In one evening, at separate times, two patients enter an Accident and Emergency Department. Each of the patients has been a victim of a knife crime. Both patients report that they have been attacked by an individual and both describe what seems to be the same person. The patients claim that the attacks were unprovoked and they did not know the attacker. The attacks happenned within a mile of each other in a busy city centre. One of the patients is happy to speak to the police and informs the Accident and Emergency staff of this. However, the other victim does not wish to have his information disclosed to the police because he does not want to be a police witness. He leaves before the police are called out.

Should the Accident and Emergency staff report both incidents to the police? Should the identity of the patients and the details of the injuries be reported?

Decision

It is generally accepted that the reporting of knife and gun crimes will be within the public interest. Accident and Emergency units should have standard procedures for informing the police that a knife crime has occurred. It should also be standard practice for staff to seek patient consent to involve the police. A knife attack may be sufficient to justify a public interest disclosure of confidential information even when consent has not been given, where it is likely to assist in the prevention, detection or prosecution of a serious crime. In this example, police could be called to interview the first person, who could then be expected to identify himself, and provide a description of the attack and the attacker, and of his injuries. If the patient refused to provide some of these details, the hospital could provide them. For the second patient it is likely to be proportionate to provide the police with details of the patient, the attacker, the attack and the patient's injuries.

Scenario 3

Following a series of complaints to a Member of Parliament from local residents, all of whom suffer a particular disease and live close to a nuclear power station, a project is set up to investigate whether the proximity to the power station could contribute to the onset of the disease. The investigation team from the Public Health observatory seeks access to confidential information within approximately two thousand paper case notes in the local hospital trust in order to discover the prevalence of relevant symptoms.

The team argues that it is not feasible to seek consent from patients within the timescales of the enquiry and that their work can be justified in the public interest.

Decision

The hospital Caldicott Guardian considers that the risk of serious harm is not sufficient to breach the confidence of thousands of patients. However she feels there is a strong public interest in the investigation. In order to minimise the potential detriment caused, she offers to assist the investigation by providing local clinical coding staff to extract relevant data from the case notes and provide it to the investigation team. Nevertheless, the data to be provided could still reveal patient identity, and so she instructs the investigation team that the information provided must be stored and processed securely, and that no identifiable patient information will be published without explicit patient consent.

■ DEMONSTRATING RECORD KEEPING WITH CHILD CONSENT

Scenario 4

Sara, aged 15, wants to accept immunisation as part of the school immunisation programme, but her mother has contacted her school to refuse consent. The school nurse discusses the benefits and risks of immunisation with Sara and forms the view that Sara is mature enough to understand the implications of having the immunisation. The nurse phones Sara's mother to try to explain that Sara is legally able to consent for herself and that having discussed the risks and benefits she wishes to go ahead. Sara's mother finally accepts that her daughter is able to make up her own mind. Even without the final agreement of Sara's mother, the immunisation could lawfully have been given, but the nurse was anxious to achieve consensus wherever possible.

Decision

The school nurse will record the account in the records, including the establishment of Sara's competency (capacity), the outcomes of the discussion with Sara's mother and the type of consent gained from Sara to allow the immunisation to go ahead. The entry will be made as near to the time of the event as possible so as to comply with keeping contemporaneous records. The record keeping in this scenario should show clearly what the school nurse did and the outcomes that were achieved. If the notes are required at a later date in a court of law they must show clearly the process of the decision-making and demonstrate the school nurse's accountability.

Crown copyright material is reproduced under the terms and conditions of the Open Government Licence (OGL).

Key references

Audit Commission (1999) *Setting the Record Straight. A Review of Progress in Health Records Services.* Audit Commission Publications, Oxford.

Department of Health (2003) *Confidentiality: NHS Code of Practice.*

Department of Health (2006) *Records Management: NHS Code of Practice.*

Department of Health (2010) *Confidentiality: Supplementary Guidance: Public Interest Disclosures.*

Dimond, B. (1998) Legal aspects of clinical supervision 2: Professional accountability. *British Journal of Nursing*, 7:8.

Glover, D. (1999) *Accountability.* Nursing Times monograph no 27. Emap Healthcare, London.

Nursing and Midwifery Council (2009) *Record Keeping: Guidance for Nurses and Midwives.*

Nursing and Midwifery Council (2009) *Guidance on Professional Conduct for Nursing and Midwifery Students.*

Nursing and Midwifery Council (2008) *The Code. Standards of Conduct, Performance and Ethics for Nurses and Midwives.*

Pennels, C. (1997) Nursing and the law: Clinical responsibility. *Professional Nurse*, 13:3. Cited in Glover, D. (1999) *Accountability.* Nursing Times monograph no 27. Emap Healthcare, London.

Pullen, I. and Loudon, J. (2006) Improving standards in clinical record keeping. *Advances in Psychiatric Treatment*, 12. http//apt.rcpsych.org/

Pyne, R. (1981) *Professional Discipline in Nursing, Midwifery and Health Visiting.* Blackwell Science, Oxford.

Tingle J. (1998) Clinical governance and record keeping: Legal issues. *British Journal of Community Nursing*, 3:8.

Useful websites

www.legislation.gov.uk/ukpga/1990/23/section/1
Access to Health Records Act 1990

www.legislation.gov.uk
Computer Misuse Act 1990

www.legislation.gov.uk/ukpga/1998/29/c
Data Protection Act 1998

www.dh.gov.uk/publicationpolicyandguidance
Department of Health (2001) National Service Framework for Older People

www.doh.uk/consent
Department of Health (2001) Seeking Consent: Working with children

www.legislation.gov.uk
Disability Discrimination Act 1995

www.hri.org
European Convention on Human Rights

www.legislation.gov.uk
Freedom of Information Act 2000

www.legislation.gov.uk
Human Fertilisation and Embryology Act 1990

www.legislation.gov.uk/ukpga/2005/9
Mental Capacity Act 2005

www.legislation.gov.uk
National Health Service Venereal Disease Regulation 1974

www.connectingforhealth.nhs.uk
NHS Connecting for Health (2011)

www.nmc-uk.org/advicebytopic/confidentiality
Nursing and Midwifery Council. Confidentiality

www.legislation.gov.uk
Race Relations Act 1976

T - #0002 - 071024 - C0 - 120/80/2 - SB - 9780273760641 - Gloss Laminatio